The Alkaline Diet Best Guide

Anneliese McMiller

Copyright © 2022 by Anneliese McMiller

All rights reserved.

No portion of this book may be reproduced in any form without written permission from the publisher or author, except as permitted by U.S. copyright law.

Contents

1. The Book — 1
2. Sme Tips — 35
3. Recipes — 47
4. My personal recipes — 57

Chapter One

The Book

Almost everybody needs to lose weight and remain fit, and however not everybody is prepared to do what will empower them lose weight. In a few other circumstances, the will is there, but the information is missing. The previous is the case most of the time anyway. It could be a prevalent saying that information is control, but information which is unapplied yields no result. Hence, it is more secure to say that information when connected is power. On your weight misfortune travel, it is imperative to know the prerequisites which can abdicate ideal comes about. With regard to alkaline slim down, it is imperative to know how the body frameworks work, what ph level involves, how to require diets which adjust the ph levels, people it is appropriate to (can anybody set out on such travel, or is it limited to a select few). These and numerous more got to be handled some time recently one sets out on such a travel, as wellbeing they say, is riches.

To remain sound, shed weight and remain fit would continuously require a few frame of obstinacy since days will emerge after you would fair need to eat anything, it would be as in spite of the fact that you woke up on the off-base side of the bed and nearly anything you choose to do may stay worthless subsequently the motivation to fling nourishment. You must get it some time recently you begin this switch that certain days like these would come and your capacity to stand up to motivation and delay satisfaction would go a long way to decide how long your travel would final. Many questions come to intellect when the subject of eat less is raised, a few individuals accept it works, others don't whereas others are Detached in spite of the fact that they would cherish to have the bodies of a few of those who guzzle a alter in their different schedules, counting what they eat.

The kidney could be a major roleplayer within the capacity of the body to direct and control the sharpness of body liquids. With this information, the French scientist Claude Bernard appeared a classical think about where he utilized rabbits as example. He found that changing the slim down of rabbits from a plant (herbivore) count calories to an creature count calories (carnivore) changed the pee from more antacid to more corrosive. Activated by this finding, he set out on more examination and dug into the chemical properties and causticity of constituents found in nourishments combusted in a calorimeter, alluded to as fiery remains. He proposed that when nourishment is metabolized, a comparative "corrosive fiery remains" or "soluble fiery remains" is cleared out within the body as those oxidized in combustion.

This speculation got refined around the 20th century by sustenance researchers. Included to their finding was the intercession within the part of adversely charged particles (anions) and emphatically charged particles (cations) in nourishment, this specific finding got the attention of nutritionists, because it gave a diverse see which had not been known some time recently at that point, on how diverse diets were anions whereas others were cations. Diets which were negatively charged (those which contained phosphate, sulfate additionally chloride) were respected as corrosive shaping diets whereas those wealthy in magnesium, calcium and potassium (cations) were regarded to be antacid shaping. This think about went on and within the conclusion, it was concluded that changing the body's pH level can offer assistance to progress your wellbeing additionally offer assistance lose weight. In case the body's causticity level is raised, it seem chance the increment of long term complications like cancer and joint pain. What the antacid diets points at doing is for you to eat nourishments which keep the pH level always more alkalinic, this moreover makes a difference improve the work of the kidney amid digestion system since the kidney would not have to be metabolize a parcel of constituents, compared to an acidic content. What does an soluble slim down mean? For the straightforward reality that there's the word "alkaline", it basically would cruel there would ought to be a connection to "acidic". These words are utilized with regard to pH levels. PH is essentially the degree of how acidic or alkalinic something is. The pH esteem for the most part ranges from 0-14. Acidic speaks to 0.0 to 6.9, impartial is at 7.0 whereas antacid or fundamental is from 7.1 to 14.0.

When talking about the antacid slim down, it is vital to get it pH and how it capacities. The blood pH run when ordinary is 7.35 to 7.45. Thus, we are able say that actually, blood is somewhat soluble or basic. It was accepted that the blood pH may be modified by the kind of nourishment a human being devours, but this has not been demonstrated by any dependable sources, in case the kind of nourishment being devoured by a individual seem modify the blood pH level, that would weaken the action of the acid-base homeostasis. Homeostasis includes the capacity of a framework or living life form to adjust its inner environment to preserve a state of consistency e.g. the capacity of warm blooded creatures to preserve a steady temperature. The same applies to human being. Acid-base homeostasis is entirely carried out by the body itself, the nourishment you take into your framework does not precisely change this, and indeed in the event that it does, it does so in negligible and transitory amount. framework does not precisely modify this, and indeed on the off chance that it does, it does so in negligible and temporal amount. The pH level of the blood is promptly reestablished by the kidneys and the respiratory framework. That negligible amount in which it does so may well be all that's required to set up a connect that there's some shape of change which occurs between the nourishment admissions and the blood pH level.

The pH

According to specialists, the correct adjust of pH within the body is by and large considered the solution for wellbeing and long life. This implies you must have a pH adjust. The nourishment you eat contains the nutrients required for typical metabolic work but after you devour nourishments without knowing the supplement substance, you remain destitute of the dietary esteem included to your body and you have got no thought in the event that you're preparing or harming your wellbeing. Side effects like stomach related afflictions, weight pick up, discouragement, tiredness, cerebral pains and a common feeling of discomfort cruel that the body is out adjust and has incessant abundance corrosiveness.

Shockingly, when indications like these appear up, the another thing would be attending to the drug store to induce a fast settle. This would as it were die down the side effects for a while and however the underlying issue still continues, and this remains more inconvenient within the long run. The complete metabolic handle is subordinate on an soluble environment. In the event that the blood pH drops underneath 6.8 or rises over 7.8, at that point there's a plausibility that death is inescapable. When the body gets to be sick, it is regularly a sign to show that the body has gotten to be as well acidic and the inside liquids within the body needs the alkalinity required to operate at its best. Once notice isn't taken in regard of these signs, at that point over time, aggravation may create and cancer gets shaped, heart maladies result conjointly diabetes comes up. To unravel this issue, it is prudent to go on an antacid eat less as your body would perform at its best and weight would be lost.

Digestion system, which alludes to the transformation of nourishment into vitality, a chemical response which breaks down strong mass is included be that as it may, these chemical responses happen very gradually and in a controlled way. Metabolic squander is remained after you've got eaten. This squander can influence the body's sharpness to an degree. This little sum of corrosive aggregation can happen from dietary awkwardness, this corrosive is labeled "metabolic corrosive" since it comes about from the body's digestion system and the digestion system of nourishment over a long time, and this would inevitably result in unremitting, low-grade metabolic acidosis which causes harms to the body. The antacid nourishments are considered to be more defensive, compared to the acidic nourishments. Nourishment moreover, can alter the pH esteem of pee. The body controls its blood pH through one of the numerous ways which incorporate excreting corrosive in pee.

Making Your Individual Arrange

The Considerations In making your individual arrange, you must put a couple of things into thought, lion's share of which is centered on information. Information engages effectiveness, the more learned on a matter you're, the more compelling you'll become. In making a individual arrange to take after, you must first Know yourself You may ponder why we are towing the way of Socrates, well, almost everything he said can be appropriate in nearly each circle of life. Within the words of Socrates, "Man, know thyself".

This small but essential statement can easily be forgotten and considered insignificant, but its importance cannot be exaggerated. In a group of humans, what they know about themselves is much more important and much more important than what others say to them. When you step into the bar and ask the bartender to give you vodka, another man comes in and orders from Hennessy. He begins to feel uneasy when the person who ordered the vodka is still linking its value to net worth. In two ways-he can shyly tilt his head and look in the opposite direction, or be overly frank and throw tantrums here and there. Those who know their value and who they are are completely aware that their value should not be tied to their wealth. With that understanding, he walks around like a good man. The same is true in this case. You need to know what you can and cannot do. In situations involving migration, you need to know that planning failures and failures are not the end of the road. Failure is just an opportunity to get a better start. It is important to get used to the diet plan you choose, rather than consider it mandatory just to punish yourself. When everything is in place, certain unexpected situations can occur. But for some reason you couldn't hit the mark. You need to schedule these days, knowing that the action you need to take is not to neglect your plans and give up, but to try again the next day. It takes a lot of time to start something and keep it faithful, especially when it comes to food, the plug of life. First off, you must know your limits and be able to test boundaries by stretching such limits, just to see how far you can go, with time, it will become second nature. Take for instance a boy who says he cannot read for 1 hour, having set such a limitation in his mind, while reading, even though he may still be interested in reading, once it gets to an hour, he finds himself packing up his books, this is simply because meditation is the law of the mind.

.. The plasticity of the brain allows such things to happen, so the brain can be stretched rather than static. Just as you can develop a habit, it can be counteracted by other habits. Knowing who you are and what you can do takes you to the fulcrum of consciousness, and you can change what you believe to gain the acquisition of your mind. You can and it will be easier with practice. Your lifestyle

Lifestyles generally play a big role in the other activities you engage in. If you try to adapt to a particular plan many times and then always fail, you may not need a fortune teller to tell you what the problem is. It doesn't really get into your lifestyle. Of course, if you're an athlete, the way you do things is different from the way taxi drivers do things, and it extends to everything related to health. Lifestyle is very important in deciding what diet you want. It may seem negligible, but it's not too far away, so such a small thing can make all the difference. Looking at your lifestyle from this angle, you can estimate the cost. You don't always have to deny yourself some of the cute tresses with cherry toppings everywhere for your lifestyle and still embark on a painstaking task like flopping. If you need to change your lifestyle, be sure to do it. Alkaline diets bring great benefits to the body not only for food, but also when performing other necessary activities at an alarming rate. One of these necessary activities is exercise. Exercise should be part of your daily life. If you don't exercise more than once a week, you won't feel well. Instead of getting on a bus or driving a car, simply walking is a form of exercise. You cannot lift weights in the gym before you can confirm that you have exercised. Simple stretching in the room is another form of exercise. The body should be taken good care of and should not be neglected in any case. This body is the only thing you will get for a long time, so there are many things to consider before making a particular decision.

Nutrients

You need to have a solid understanding of how such things work, what kind of food should I eat? Knowing the right nutrients allows you to prepare your own meals rather than relying solely on information from the internet or elsewhere. Of course, you can do some validation, but it only helps to supplement what you already know, and for those who don't know what to do or exactly what to take. It will be very difficult. Knowledge of the various nutrients remains the basis for being able to adjust your diet to suit you as you lose weight and become healthier. As mentioned above, a negatively charged diet (containing phosphates, sulfates, and chlorides) is considered an acid-forming diet, and a diet high in magnesium, calcium, and potassium (cations) is an alkali-forming diet. Was considered. It is important to know the food class and some of its ingredients. There are seven major classes of nutrients: carbohydrates, fats, fiber, minerals, proteins, vitamins and water. These nutrients are divided into micronutrients and macronutrients. Major nutrients include carbohydrates, proteins, and fats, which are energy sources. Water and fiber are also major nutrients, but they do not produce energy. Micronutrients are essentially minerals and vitamins.

Carbohydrates – Classified as monosaccharides, disaccharides, or polysaccharides, depending on the number of sugar units they contain. They are made up of most of the foods such as rice, pasta and bread. Carbohydrates are not essential nutrients and do not necessarily have to be ingested by humans. The brain is the body's largest sugar consumer and uses large amounts of glucose. When glucose isn't enough to do that business, it switches to fat.

Fat-There are saturated and unsaturated fats, and unsaturated fats are considered to be healthier than saturated fats. These unsaturated fats, such as vegetable oils, come from plants, and saturated fats come from animals. Humans have two fatty acids that are very important and should be included in every diet: omega-3 and omega-6. Dietary Fiber Dietary fiber belongs to the group of carbohydrates and is divided into insoluble fiber and soluble fiber. Soluble fiber is a fiber that humans can digest and provides some calories to the body.

Whole grains, fruits, and even vegetables are excellent sources of dietary fiber. Fiber helps reduce the risk of colon cancer

Proteins – These are components of the body structure of many animals and make up the enzymes that control reactions throughout the body. Proteins are composed of amino acids that break down nitrogen and sometimes sulfur. A diet containing sufficient amounts of amino acids (required). Excess amino acids from proteins are converted to glucose and used as fuel throughout gluconeogenesis.

Minerals-Dietary minerals are the inorganic elements needed by living organisms. There are macro minerals and trace minerals. Macrominerals contain calcium, which is essential for cardiovascular and muscle health. It is essential for bone formation and supports the structure and function of blood cells in the body. Sauces include dairy products, leafy vegetables and broccoli. Other macrominerals include magnesium, chloride ions, phosphorus, potassium and sodium. Trace elements include manganese, iron and molybdenum. Calcium: You can't talk about developing strong bones without mentioning calcium. Calcium is necessary for growth, is necessary for all humans, and an alkaline diet must be rich in calcium. Most of the body's calcium is found in bones and teeth. Calcium is also needed to facilitate communication between the brain and all other parts of the body. Its role in cardiovascular function and muscle movement cannot be ignored. Calcium is naturally present in some foods and can be added to certain products. Potassium: Studies show that the human body needs at least 100 milligrams of potassium daily to support growth and development. This potassium is found in alkaline diets and is mostly fully incorporated. It reduces the risk of stroke, protects the body from loss of muscle mass, maintains bone density and reduces kidney stones. Their main goals include adjusting fluid balance and controlling electrical activity in the heart and muscles. Potassium is needed to maintain acid-base balance in the body and counteracts the effects of sodium.

. When potassiumrich foods are consumed, the alkaline environment in the body is maintained, unlike in acidosis, which is triggered by a diet full of acidifying foods which includes meat, processed grains etc. acidosis also causes nitrogen excretion, and a loss in bone mineral density follows. Potassium is contained in foods such as fresh leafy greens, avocados, tomatoes, potatoes, and beans. In the events of processing foods, the amount of dietary potassium is reduced. Iron: In hemoglobin and myoglobin, iron is the main oxygen carrier. It absolutely requires its presence for proper oxygenation of blood and cells. This mineral is also involved in electrochemical reactions in the brain, is an iron-containing enzyme that is part of the Krebs circuit, and also helps eliminate toxins such as hydrogen hydrogen, which helps in energy production. The body needs about 6 to 20 milligrams of iron daily, which can lead to hair loss, nervousness, and cognitive dysfunction if not ingested adequately. Zinc: It plays as important a role as white blood cells and helps the body fight viral and bacterial infections. The role of zinc in regulating cell regeneration cannot be exaggerated, and it is also necessary to regulate the treatment of other important alkaline minerals such as calcium and magnesium. Zinc helps fight diseases such as osteoporosis and osteoarthritis associated with mineral deficiency as a result of acid-base imbalance. Magnesium: Magnesium plays an important role in over 300 enzymatic reactions in the human system. Above all, it promotes muscle and nerve function, helps regulate blood pressure, and also supports the immune system. This magnesium is found in most alkaline diets, so it is best to choose such a level of diet. The adult human body contains about 25 grams of magnesium, and the skeletal system stores about 5060% of it. The rest is contained in soft tissues, muscles and body fluids. Alkaline diets are rich in magnesium, so the best way to get enough magnesium in your diet is to eat an alkaline diet. Eat at least 100 milligrams (mg) daily. The other microminerals that exist are iron and zinc, but people need them in small amounts. There are clearly several benefits to getting enough of this mineral.

Bone Health: Magnesium is essential for many proper functions of the body. Therefore, you need to get enough magnesium to protect your body from infections such as chronic and cardiovascular diseases, bone damage, Alzheimer's disease, migraine, and type 2 diabetes. It also promotes healthy bone growth and formation. Studies show that higher bone density is associated with magnesium as well as calcium, and postmenopausal women have a lower risk of osteoporosis. Improving bone density can be direct or indirect and helps regulate calcium and vitamin D levels. A basic diet promotes magnesium absorption.

Diabetes: A magnesium-rich diet is associated with a reduced risk of diabetes (type 2). This is because magnesium plays an important role in glucose regulation and insulin metabolism. Several studies have reported that most people with diabetes are low in magnesium. Insulin resistance is associated with magnesium deficiency, magnesium deficiency exacerbates insulin resistance, and insulin resistance leads to lower magnesium levels. Taking magnesium supplements may improve insulin sensitivity in people with low magnesium levels. Cardiovascular Health: To maintain the health of the heart muscle, including the heart, certain requirements must be met, one of which is the high levels of magnesium in the body. Magnesium plays an important role in the proper functioning of the heart. A magnesium-deficient body also has a role at the cellular level and may increase the risk of heart disease. Magnesium deficiency has been identified in people with heart failure and can exacerbate clinical outcomes. Magnesium helps stabilize the heart, and people who take some form of magnesium after treating the heart tend to be much better off. Magnesium can be used as part of the treatment of congestive heart failure to reduce the risk of arrhythmias. Studies show that increasing magnesium intake reduces the risk of stroke. Foods rich in magnesium can also help lower blood pressure

Migraine: Magnesium deficiency affects neurotransmitters and limits angioplasty. This can lead to migraine headaches, and magnesium therapy can help prevent or relieve headaches. Low levels of magnesium in the blood are associated with a high incidence of migraine in people. Therefore, magnesium administration helps fight migraine headaches. Vitamin-Vitamin D is also an important part of an alkaline diet. Vitamin D, along with calcium and magnesium, promotes healthy bone growth, which helps prevent osteoporosis and strengthens bones. With the exception of Vitamin D, all other vitamins are essential nutrients and are necessary in the diet for good health. An important factor associated with weight loss and an alkaline diet is the fact that bone mass must be taken into account to avoid certain illnesses such as osteoporosis.

Certain conditions such as osteoporosis

Osteoporosis: Osteoporosis literally means porous bone. The disease reduces bone quality and density. As the body grows, some adjustment is needed and bone quality becomes important. Some bones become porous and weak, increasing the risk of fractures. This bone loss occurs quietly and poses no threat at first unless one knows what is happening, but over time the effects begin to be felt. Osteoporosis is closely related to age and is said to reduce estrogen production and change the structure of regenerated bone when women reach the age of menopause. In people suffering from osteoporosis, bone loss tends to outweigh the growth of new bone, making the bone porous and prone to fractures. Osteoporosis-related fractures most commonly occur in the spine, wrists, and hips. With age, both men and women are more likely to experience these hip and spinal fractures. The consequences of fractures of the spine and hips are extremely detrimental and can lead to severe back pain, short stature, and deformities. In addition to age, which plays a major role in osteoporosis, dietary nutrients also play an important role. A diet rich in calcium, magnesium and phosphorus is important. In addition to calcium, you also need vitamin D. This Vitamin D helps absorb calcium from certain products. The roles that calcium plays are:

Bone: The main component of bone development is calcium. Calcium maintains bones even after a person's growth has stopped. Calcium helped delay the loss of bone density that is naturally associated with the aging process. Bone density is lost more often in postmenopausal women than in younger people. Regular intake of calcium helps to strengthen these bones. Muscle contraction: Calcium in the body regulates muscle contraction. As long as the nerves stimulate the muscles, calcium is released. Calcium in protein also helps muscle contraction. When calcium is excreted from the muscles by the body, the muscles expand.

Cardiovascular system: The benefits of an alkaline diet rich in calcium also affect blood clotting. The coagulation step contains a variety of chemicals, including calcium. It also helps maintain the heart muscle. It has been found that an increase in calcium intake may be associated with a decrease in blood pressure. Calcium plays a role alongside enzymes, but without calcium certain enzymes do not work properly. Calories

In a bid to lose weight, the things to embark on and the paraphernalia needed must be properly understood to avoid any form of mishap. So, what are calories? In order to lose weight, fewer calories must be taken into the system when compared to the number of calories which is being burned. Counting or taking note of your calorie intake is an important way of tracking weight gain, and with intermittent fasting, it becomes easier. Calories is a term borrowed from physics. In science, calories are a measure of energy, and when used in relation to nutrition, they are used to measure the energy content of foods. Food calories can be defined as the amount of energy required to raise the temperature of a kilogram of water by 1 degree Celsius. Calories have an indispensable function for the human body and are used in daily life. When you say that you have consumed a lot of energy, you are losing a lot of calories. Calories are spent talking, breathing, walking, and even thinking. Calories that are not used to perform a function are stored as fat. Therefore, if you eat more consistently than you burn, you will gain weight. You may think calories do not matter and that counting calories is a waste of time but as regards your weight, a whole lot matters and calories is inclusive. This has been proven time and again in some studies referred to as overfeeding studies. In studies such as these, people are asked to deliberately overfeed and the impact on their weight and health is measured. Through these studies, it has been noted that the more calories people take in with relatively less calorie burn, the more weight they gain. This means that to prevent weight gain and also lose weight, limiting your intake and also counting your calorie poses as an effective method. The amount of calories you need depends on specific factors such as gender, age, weight, and even the level of activity you enjoy on a daily basis. For example, a 25-year-old man who fasts intermittently and goes to the gym needs more calories than a 54-year-old woman who does not exercise regularly.

"Diet quality has a big impact on how you lose fat and how you feel good, but it's important to keep in mind that foods have different calorie content. For example, 150 calories of broccoli are good for your health. It has different effects. Up to 150 calories of french fries. This is because your overall diet and the type of food you put into your system affect how you grow and develop. The effects of different foods on hormones, hunger, etc. are different and the amount of calories burned can vary significantly. It is important to maintain a high quality diet with foods from minimally processed plants and animals. Knowing the ingredients and functions of these nutrients will help you know exactly what to eat. Taking the right alkaline diet will eventually suit whatever purposes for which you decided to change your diet style to alkaline dieting

A lot of diets have become popular for some reason. Already, there are lots of testimonies on alkaline dieting, even from celebrities, it has gained a lot of recognition as a result of its transformation on the body, a little of it has been stated earlier. There are quite a lot of benefits of alkaline dieting; antiaging effect will obviously be a part of it because there will be an increase in insulin sensitivity and there will also be weight loss which is related to a reduction in the intake of calorie.

According to recent studies, a diet induced weight loss plan was followed and it led to about a 70% weight gain. Finding the weightloss plan which works best for you is imperative.

Eating everything you can get is definitely not the best way to go. Even people who are not on a diet will eat unhealthy foods. If you decide to switch to an alkaline diet, it is best to carry out your plan completely. It can be difficult anyway, but in the long run you'll find that it was all for your own benefit.

Principles of Personal Planning

This includes scheduling by phone or simply writing it down on a piece of paper and sticking it on the kitchen wall to get an accurate picture of what to eat at any time of the day. .. More on breakfast, lunch, supper, and other healthy snacks in the next chapter. For some reason, even after taking an alkaline diet for a while and following your routine on a daily basis, you may still experience undesired results. It is important to know that a process always exists. You need to learn to enjoy the process. The growth process takes time. Everything else, nothing falls from the sky. You can't keep your weight away, just as you didn't want it alone. It took action and took time. No one goes to the gym and in 3 days all muscle mass comes out in the right place. It takes time and the same thing happens here. You need to understand the process and learn to appreciate small progress. Even if it looks small, it's something worth celebrating to make as little progress as following your daily menu. It is such a small celebration that leads to the biggest. So enjoy the process, it will be a long ride.

You may decide to start with a once-daily alkaline diet. For example, eat a fruit breakfast or vegetable juice for breakfast, take regular customers for lunch and dinner, and take time to increase this to two alkaline meals. One day, then you were finally able to interrupt your meal three times a day. If you make a mistake and don't feel sick, don't forget to start over. In your personal plan, there are some principles you should keep in mind, including these in your menu plan will save you a lot of stress.

Always consume a wide variety of fresh, high-quality, whole foods.

If you can get your hands on organically grown or biodynamically grown produce, that would be fantastic because this is the foundation of alkaline diet. You can't go on a diet of alkaline foods if you're still eating a lot of processed foods. Vegetables and fruits, gently toasted nut and seed mixes, sprouts of grain and bean sprouts and vegetable juices are all excellent sources of alkaline meals that can be consumed. Digestibility is aided by the enzymes included in certain foods.

You must consume a wide variety of whole foods in order to reap the benefits. If the digestive system is damaged, stressed, or otherwise affected, the body is more likely to become sensitive to the same foods as a result of eating the same thing over and over again. It is essential to broaden one's horizons when it comes to the options available. Before experimenting with new flavours, be sure you understand the nutritional value of each of the ingredients.

Alkaline-Forming Foods should make up 60% to 80% of your diet.

Never take for granted that you already know what's in your meal; always do a double-check to make sure you're getting the most bang for your calorie buck. Consume foods high in alkaline constituents to maintain a healthy pH balance. At least 80% of your food should be alkaline, which will aid in weight loss. The importance of taking care of your physical health cannot be overstated if you are to attain the full potential of your existence. Rather of looking for quick remedies if your body's immune system has been impaired, you should take necessary efforts to repair it by following an alkaline diet.

3) Consume Foods That Support Your Immune System

What your immune system reacts to must be known; this requires going to the hospital and having tests done on your body to find out if you have certain conditions like ulcers or allergies. Your body will not react to the meals you eat with this information. The metabolism speeds up when alkaline foods are swapped for acid-producing ones and nonreactive foods are consumed by persons who are overweight or obese. Underweight persons, on the other hand, gain weight because a healthy diet boosts protein production and repair.

When it comes to carbohydrates, you should eat 60% to 70% plant-based, complex carbs, 20% protein, and 20% healthy fat.

In order to get the most out of alkaline dieting, this divide has been found to be an efficient method of alkaline diet. The body's energy requirements can be met by consuming a diet high in complex carbohydrates. The following ratios are suggested.

Ratios to Use:

Whole food (plant-based) complex carbs make up about 60% to 70% of the calories consumed.

a protein-rich diet provides 15–20% of total daily caloric intake

15% to 20% of your calories should come from healthy fats (including plenty of omega-3 fats)

Complex Carbohydrates from Plant Foods:

Unless your immune system is disposed to this and your doctor has confirmed this, your alkaline eating plan must be rich in complex carbohydrates, which include vegetables, whole grains, legumes (beans, peas, and lentils), as well as seasonings, spices, and herbs. 65% to 70% of your food consumption should be made up of these.

High-Quality Meat

On this one, there should be no debate: proteins should make up roughly 15% of your entire calorie consumption. For the majority of people, a daily protein intake of 45 to 55 grammes suffices. Organic eggs and dairy products, as well as fish like mackerel, sardines, salmon, herring, and even tuna, can all be good sources of protein. There are many more sources of protein that you can include in your diet: nuts, seeds, blue-green algae, nutritious yeasts, and sprouts. It is possible to make beneficial "complimentary proteins" by combining grains with beans or gains with dairy. If you're pregnant, your protein needs may be higher than they otherwise would be. Keeping your doctor informed and working closely with him to provide you with the correct advice is essential if you are recovering from a chronic condition, exercising frequently, or have any other special demands.

Healthy fats:

Your daily calorie intake should include at least 15% of your calories from fat. The omega-3 essential fats, which are vital for energy synthesis, protein manufacturing and tissue repair, should be your primary emphasis. Fresh nuts and seeds, cold-pressed organic oils, safflower, walnut, flaxseed, sesame, peanut, and pure deep-sea fish oils are the most common food sources of protective omega-3 essential fats.

Black currant, grape seed, and primrose oil are further possible sources. Omega-3 supplements must be free of contamination or oxidation during processing before they can be used.

Complete proteins can be found in the following foods:

Plant proteins lack some necessary amino acids, but animal protein contains all of them. You'll be able to get what you need if you combine two foods based on their amino acid content. In the absence of an essential amino acid, cooked beans and brown rice are both incomplete proteins, whereas consumed together, they provide a complete protein source and complement one another. A "complete protein" can be made by combining these foods:

Been-and-rice bowls

Grains and legumes

Dairy-enriched grains

Nuts, seeds, and legumes are incorporated into dairy products.

As agriculture itself, the practise of ingesting complementary proteins has been around for a long time. Many modern meals, such as the following, have reflected and shown these influences:

- Corn, beans, and rice are included in this category.

- Indian dal with rice

- Chopped walnuts on brown rice

garbanzo bean meals made with bulgur wheat

- Almond butter spread on whole wheat toast

Trans fats and hydrogenated oils should be completely avoided at all costs

Trans fats are harmful to the body regardless of how undetectable they appear to be. Most of the time, the body treats them as if they were natural saturated fats, but they are actually hazardous. In foetal tissues, they can cause long-term problems with cell membrane function since they cross the placenta. It is unfortunate that these Trans-fats are so prevalent; they may be found in everything from fried food to baked goods to brand cooking oils.

Learn to use "expeller-pressed" oils like olive, grape seed, coconut, and peanut oil as well as "strange" oils like avocado, almond, and mustard seed in your cooking. You must avoid solid cooking fats such as margarine, hydrogenated vegetable oils, and lard in order to avoid Tran's fat and hydrogenated oil. Deep-fried dishes would also have to go.

Hydrogenated oil, which interferes with liver enzymes, is strongly linked to elevated cholesterol levels. These synthetic oils can also impair immunological function and have been linked to the development of some types of cancerous tumours.

Incorporate Foods and Drinks with Fermented (Cultured) Probiotic Cultures

The term "probiotic" refers to anything that enhances the quality of life. Your feeding plan would have to incorporate cultured foods. Even if you don't like the concept at first, you should change your opinion about it because of the potential health benefits. You should also take a range of supplements to avoid becoming dependent on a single one. A healthy gastrointestinal tract contains the microorganisms that keep the body and immune system in check. Maintaining a healthy body and immune system is made easier by the presence of these microorganisms. Deficiencies in helpful bacteria can be caused by a variety of factors, including malnutrition, stress, disease, and the use of antibiotics, all of which allow pathogens to flourish and eventually take over. Probiotics are necessary if we are to successfully colonise and take over the stomach with healthy microorganisms. To get the most probiotics, it is best to eat or drink probiotic-enriched foods and beverages like yoghurt. It's possible to take probiotic supplements if you can't get your hands on probiotic-rich foods and beverages. Probiotic-rich meals and beverages include the following.

Foods and beverages that are high in probiotics

- Kombucha is a type of tea that has been fermented.

- Kefir is a type of fermented milk.

Live cultures can be found in both dairy and non-dairy yoghurts.

fermented cabbage is another name for sauerkraut.

fermented cabbage that is prominent in the Korean diet known as "kimchi"

Soybeans are fermented, and the result is tempeh.

It's better to freeze-dry microalgae.

- Miso soup Hatcho

The Pickles

Tobacco: Olives

Noodles, or natto (a fermented soybean)

6) Make sure you're getting enough fibre and fluids.

Drinking a lot of water, at least eight glasses a day, aids the body's metabolism of food. Traditional civilizations that routinely drink water have been found to be free of some degenerative diseases that plague the typical human. Their diets also include a lot of whole, living foods, which provide a good source of fibre. The amount of fibre they consume on a daily basis is estimated to be between 40 and 100 grammes, whereas those afflicted by degenerative diseases consume less than 10 grammes. It is suggested that adults consume 40 grammes of fibre each day. Fiber's "roughage," which adds weight and softness to the stool, helps keep it moving along more quickly. During this period, a person eats food and then throws it away. In order to keep the body clean and clear, eating a diet high in fibre encourages regular and effective waste elimination. Cleanliness and clarity in the body mean that harmful waste is less likely to be reabsorbed into the circulation of the body Toxic waste is less likely to be reabsorbed into circulation if our bodies are clean and clear.

A healthy transit period spans from about 11 to 18 hours, which reduces the possibility for harmful bacteria and yeast to take hold of the body.

Water's Importance

In order to stay healthy, you need to drink a lot of water, especially if you're on a fiber-heavy diet. Water aids fiber's ability to do its work by flushing wastes out of the body. In addition, the body's systems rely on water to function. Adding a glass of pure water for every 6-8 ounces of caffeinated beverages is essential when following an alkaline diet. You should drink at least one 9-ounce glass of water every eight times daily. Taking a 30-minute break from drinking water prior to and following meals is essential for the body's digestion. These periods necessitate the consumption of room temperature or even hot water, which may sound strange and worrisome but cold water actually slows down digestion, so you'll have to get used to not drinking it. Fresh lemon, lime, or ginger juice, as well as other alkaline-boosting liquids, are excellent digestion aides and water flavour enhancers. As a result, after ingesting them, water takes on a more flavorful quality.

One cannot overstate the importance of water and the part it plays in the body; water is a need, and it is expected that you consume plenty of it. Sometimes, it may look like you have had enough but most times, you actually have not.

7) Make an effort to eat a more balanced diet.

Alkaline dieting requires an ability to mix and match foods in order to produce nutritious meals…. Digestive and general health can be greatly affected by a variety of meal combinations. There needs to be a careful consideration of the best approach to combine the food. One of the most significant aspects of eating a well-balanced diet is mastering the skill of combining nutritious foods. Once you've mastered this skill and the method of starting the operation cautiously, you'll be better prepared to face the difficulties that come your way. The digestive system will experience less wear and tear when this is correctly understood and the combo is at its finest. It's important to pay special attention to food pairings if you suffer from digestive issues such as heartburn or bloating.

You must have correct understanding about your current health issues in order to create and construct a menu that will keep you from deteriorating. Compatibility and simplicity are the most crucial factors to consider while putting together a nutritious meal. While these directions or guidelines are clear, it's also important to explore healthy food combining because it isn't a one-size-fits all, and you may be suffering from a sickness that wasn't mentioned in this article. To prevent further harm to your health, it is recommended that you first see your doctor and then make your decisions based on the results of that visit.

The benefits of an alkaline diet are obvious: it provides everything you need to maintain good health.

Recipes for a hearty breakfast.

You can pick and choose from a range of recipes in this section. This collection of alkaline-friendly dishes will show you that you don't have to eat the same thing all the time if you want to stick with it.

If you're one of those people who can't figure out exactly what to eat for breakfast, you may end up eating the opposite of what you're supposed to, while others eat the same thing they're supposed to have for lunch or supper (skipping breakfast is totally wrong, according to studies, it is more important than lunch or even dinner.) The quality of a person's health is strongly linked to the amount of breakfast they eat. Breakfast is the most important meal of the day, and skipping it is a recipe for catastrophe. Whether or whether you're on an alkaline diet can have an impact on your energy, weight gain, and ageing process.

An alkaline breakfast can seem unattainable, but it is possible to have an alkaline diet and they can be produced effortlessly.

This section provides step-by-step instructions for preparing the various ingredients. You'll be drooling for more of these dinners!

Change your breakfast, and you change your life is a popular adage that couldn't be more accurate. Adapting a new morning routine can transform your life.

Chapter Two

Sme Tips

A look at each one and how it affects us in ways we don't even know about.

Whether you like it or not, skipping breakfast will make you overweight, sluggish, and depressed in the long term.

A perilous path opens up the instant you decide to stop eating breakfast altogether. Even when you're asleep your metabolism is sped up significantly (some people do not know this). You'll find that your body's metabolism slows to a crawl after a 7- to 10-hour fast since it's in such desperate need of nutrition. There is an instantaneous vicious cycle that begins: Your cells begin feeding on your body in order to get the nutrients they so desire, and over time, your body trains itself not to expect anything in the morning, this causes a much slower metabolism as your body shifts into a different mode to compensate for the hunger. For energy, it eventually clings to whatever fat it can get its hands on.

An imbalance in your blood sugar and energy levels will lead you to overeat and make poor eating decisions. When you binge, your blood sugar and energy levels are sent into a tizzy, which is bad for your health in the long run. Breakfast aids in the smooth and efficient movement of the metabolic process. It keeps you steady and prevents you from making poor food combinations and selections.

Second-worst breakfast: the hurried breakfast (also known as the let's just eat something, no matter how little there is in our stomachs)

On the way out the door or worse still on the way to work, you grab whatever you can find, even if it's a bottle of beer, since you're in a hurry. Consider the following items: a sausage roll, a piece of toast, and a bagel. Numerous other options are devoid of any kind of energising effect. To make matters worse, some of us continue to buy items while driving without researching where they came from or how they were created, resulting in further digestive system damage.

The (Low) standard acidic breakfast in the West

You're familiar with the ins and outs of a standard western breakfast, right? Bacon, sausage, cereal, toast, eggs, jam, orange juice, milk, toast, and syrup are all included. Everything on this list will deplete your energy and then set off a chain reaction that will lead to dangerously high blood sugar levels and other health problems.

You may not be getting enough sleep on the train to work because you're eating the incorrect kind of breakfast. All of your mornings could be spent doing something physical, wouldn't it be wonderful? An alkaline diet can assist you in achieving your goals in this area.

Amylopectin A, a starch in grains, can cause a wide range of health problems if consumed at this time of the day. This carbohydrate raises blood sugar levels and increases them. Sugar levels rise, and then drop, leaving no energy and an unnatural desire for sweets or anything else that could possibly bring you back to where you were before you spiked your blood sugar.

A study found that individuals were fed a diet containing 70% amylopectin, while a control group was offered a diet that included no amylopectin. According to the study's findings, participants in the amylopectin group had the greatest glucose and insulin responses of any group tested. Insulin levels are increased, which causes inflammation in the digestive system, such as leaky gut syndrome.

After each meal, the amylopectin group showed higher glucose and insulin responses. Why do you think this is? Inflammation, fat storage in the organs, leaky gut, and other health problems are all linked to high insulin levels over time. For those experiencing hormone imbalance or health problems, cutting back on grains may be a smart place to begin your journey toward wellness.

Eggs, toast, milk, and other morning staples may seem like the end of the world, but you'd be surprised to learn that there are still a number of other delicious options out there.

As an experiment, imagine waking up at 6 a.m. every day for the next month. When you have more time on your hands, what would you do with it? Maybe you've been attempting to get up and out of bed earlier and earlier, but it hasn't worked. Perhaps you'd like to spend more time at the gym or with your family. So, when you wake up at 6 a.m. every day, just write down what you'd like to do.

One of the finest things that can happen to you is the gift of energy and time that you receive from waking up early.

It's important not to put too much pressure on yourself while starting a new diet plan; the process of changing diet plans takes time, so be patient and make the necessary changes at your own pace. An alkaline, nutrient-rich breakfast is the goal of this diet; it will keep you awake, aware, and in good spirits.

Ahead of you, here's the first.

First, there's a vegan scramble with scrambled tofu and tomatoes.

Ingredients

285 grammes of tofu (Regular firm).

For this recipe, you can use either olive oil or coconut oil (approximately 1 Tablespoon in size).

Tomatoes, at least two

baby spinach, about two large handfuls

1 rocket/arugula leaf, chopped

12 onion, browned (or red if you fancy)

12 of a red chilli pepper

Add a dash of turmeric

Black pepper ground to a fine powder

Salt from the Himalayas or the sea

A dash of basil is all that is needed.

a few sprigs of cilantro or coriander

Cayenne pepper can be added for a kick.

Getting Ready

This is a cinch to put together, and it's ready in a flash. Simply crumble the tofu into a bowl with your hands. The onion should be chopped and fried fast, while the pepper should be diced and fried as well. Then, in the bowl, squeeze the tofu with your hands. Toss the diced tomatoes with the tofu, spinach, and a dash of turmeric in a bowl. After grinding your pepper and adding salt, the next step is to cook the tofu until it's done. Just before you remove the dish from the heat, add some basil leaves, the rocket, and coriander and serve it with a touch of pepper.

To accompany it, you may serve it with toasted sprouted bread and some baby spinach. Oh, the splendour! The two of you would get along great.

It's the fat-rich, fulfilling, and mouthwatering way to start the day.

You may eat this meal once a week, and it's good for your skin and your body in general because it contains vital fatty acids. This diet can be considered a "transitional" one. This dinner is delicious and filling.

You can drink it with any non-dairy milk you like, or even with no milk at all if you have some on hand (you must not take it with any milk at all, you may decide to take it with yoghurt and a half apple). This dinner is essentially a reward for your own pleasure. Making almond milk is a rather simple process. Bulk dry mix can be prepared in a large quantity and then stored in an airtight container for weeks, making it easy to access anytime you have a need for it.

Ingredients for the dish

It contains organic oats (which are inherently gluten-free but may contain traces of gluten if processed with wheat). If you have celiac disease, you should use gluten-free oats.)

Pumpkin seeds can be found in a little container.

chia seeds, about a tablespoon

Almonds, unroasted and unprocessed, in small amounts

You can also use ground flax, almond, or any other nut/seed in place of the LSA mixture.

Pumpkin seeds in a small handful

chia seed teaspoon

Milk of your choice: Almond or rice

These can be served on their own or as an accompaniment to the meal, but they work best when taken together.

A coconut yoghurt

Sliced figs (fresh ones)

Getting Ready

It's a breeze to put this together! If you don't have access to LSA milk, use any 'meal/ground' that you prefer or can get your hands on, and then combine everything and serve with milk. Regardless of where a health food store is located, there is a product that can work with this, such as flax or ground almonds.

Many people believe that this diet is ideal for the winter since it is rich in nutrients, keeps you warm, and fills you up. Full amino acid range, alkaline minerals, manganese, magnesium (which promotes bone density), iron, vitamin b2 and fibre are all included in this comprehensive protein package (which is totally necessary in all alkaline diets) This warming, satisfying, and nutrient-packed alkaline diet breakfast is ideal for the onset of winter.

Quinoa is a sure bet because it offers so much goodness in such a small package. It's quick to make, delicious, and provides you an energy boost all at once. To top it all off, the combination of fibre, carbohydrates, and proteins ensures that you'll have plenty of energy and be satisfied until your next meal comes around!

3. Breakfast Warmer Quinoa and Apple

Ingredients in the recipe

½ cup of quinoa

A single apple

2/3 of an orange

Cinnamon

a spoonful of organic coconut oil.

Dried cranberries, seeds, and nuts are optional.

Preparation: Rinse the quinoa in a sieve and add around 50% more water than the quinoa, i.e., for 2 cups of quinoa, add 2.5 cups of water. Follow the instructions on the quinoa package for the rest of the preparation. Boil it for about 15 minutes and let it to cool.

The apple is grated and cooked for an additional 30 seconds as you near the end of the 15-minute cooking period (it would be easier if you grate it already so you do not waste anymore time in grating). As a finishing touch, a bit of lemon juice is squeezed into the mixture. Serve with a dash of cinnamon and a drizzle of coconut oil, if desired. Finally, you've completed your task! A scrumptious dinner.

Dried cranberries can be added if desired, but they must be added right before the apple is chopped. Coconut yoghurt, almonds, and seeds are other good options for toppings.

Besides the fact that it correctly nourishes the body, the advantages of this diet include its filling properties, outstanding taste, and smooth, creamy texture. Fresh, raw alkaline vegetables are also included in your daily servings. I've never seen anything like this.

4. Alkaline Power Shake with Avocado

Ingredients for a recipe

It calls for one cucumber.

Tomatoes 2

A single avocado

1 serving of spinach, roughly 1 cup

1 lime, cut in half

12-teaspoon organic and gluten-free vegetable stock 50 ml filtered warm water

Extra leaves are entirely optional (lettuce, Kate etc.) Herbs and spices (basil, parsley and coriander) are included in this dish (ginger, turmeric, cumin)

Preparation: Wash the cucumber, avocado, tomato, and pepper well for the purpose of your well-being.

Place the avocado and the stock in a blender and process until they form a paste. Remove from the mixer and serve immediately. A blender would be the following step, in which high-water-content materials would be added and pulverised. The lime and supplements can now be added to the spinach, and the mixture should be completely blended before the spinach is finished.

Serve in a large glass so that you can finish everything.

Those additional optionals aren't actually necessary, but if you have them and enjoy using them, you can include them. Also, make sure you can experiment with these items on your own, because you never know what you'll discover. Just don't add fruit.

Chapter Three

Recipes

Almond milk that has not been pasteurised

Here's how to make almond milk, which we addressed in relation to a particular diet.

All you need to do for almond milk is to make sure your milk is as pure, dairy-free, and unrefined as possible. This takes care of a lot of issues. Your almond milk must be healthy and alkaline and not laden with sweets, hormones, or any other substances that appear lovely but are actually harmful to the body, such as preservatives and additives.

Ingredients:

Almond flour, 1 cup

3-cup hydration

a vanilla bean, with the seeds extracted

For the first and most crucial step, you must soak the almonds in water for at least eight hours before blending them with 3 cups of fresh water in a blender. Blend in the vanilla bean at this point to complete the mixture. With a cheesecloth or any other strainer, you'll be able to get your hands on fresh almond milk in no time!

Refrigeration is the best place to keep it. The worry of needing to prepare another one every three days or every time you want to eat your alkaline muesli would be alleviated if you made a huge batch. When creating almond milk, there are numerous methods available, but I believe it's preferable to keep things simple rather than complicate them further. Almond milk made with this recipe is the finest I've found so far.

Bacon and egg dishes

It's impossible to go a day without a slice of French toast. The most efficient and cost-effective way to make French toast is to learn the best technique. If you follow this recipe, you're guaranteed to reap the benefits on your health!

Ingredients for a recipe

Bread, brown, six slices

2 ovaries

0.5 litres of milk.

1 tablespoon of cinnamon powder

12 tsp. of salt, if desired

The vanilla extract is 1 teaspoon.

Nutmeg in a quarter teaspoon

Steps

You should begin by whisking together all of the ingredients in a large bowl until smooth.

Dip the bread in the egg mixture and allow it to soak on all sides.

Once you've done that, heat a small amount of oil in a small saucepan on a low heat.

Cook the bread until golden on both sides, about a minute or two.

Serve hot, with a pat of butter on top.

7. Pancakes with Apples

In order to make apple pancakes that are full of flavour and taste, follow these directions. You can never go wrong with apple pancakes.

The instructions for making the dish.

12 cup of all purpose flour

1 tsp. of ground cinnamon powder

Whisking a single egg

A third of a cup of milk

2 red apples, grated

2 teaspoons cooking oil

1 kiwifruit peeled

Just a few blueberries.

½ cup low-fat frozen yoghurt

Getting Ready

Take an apple and a bowl, and carefully combine the two. The next step is to add some milk and an egg. Whisk the mixture constantly until it is completely smooth.

Add a little oil to the frying pan and heat it up. Don't forget to keep the thermostat on a low setting.

Fill a large container halfway with water and then pour in the mixture.

In the pan, the apple is added.

Wait for it to cook. Two minutes should be plenty time for this.

They should be made into separate batches.

Serving suggestion: Blueberries, kiwis, and yoghurt.

8. Breakfast Salad with Avocados

The Mexican salad is one of the best in the world, with a wide variety of textures and flavours. Additionally, it has been shown to aid with weight loss.

The ingredients for this dish are listed below.

2 taco shells

Tofu in a half-pack

A single avocado

Fruit of the Pink Kind:

The equivalent of about ten almonds

Spinach in the amount of 4 ounces

Chilli sauce in a teaspoon

Tomatoes 2

Red onion, half

2/3 of an orange

Getting Ready

Oven-warm the tortillas.

To bake them, preheat the oven to 350°F and bake for 10 minutes.

Chop the tofu, tomatoes, onions, and other ingredients together on one side before adding the chilli sauce.

Put it in the fridge for a few hours before serving.

The avocado, almonds, and grapefruit are next to be chopped.

Place them carefully over the bowl after you've combined them.

Apply some fresh lemon juice to the top of the cake.

9. The symbiotic relationship between the various ingredients. Crispy Sprouts on the Side

If you're looking for a way to eat more vegetables, this mixed sprout salad is an excellent option. The flavour is also out of this world. Sprouts can be eaten raw or cooked, and they are a good source of fibre, vitamins, and minerals.

The following are the ingredients in this dish:

shoots of fenugreek

(half a cup of)

Cabbage with a reddish hue (one half cup)

Only a tiny radish was consumed.

(You'll be slicing it very thinly.)

or arugula, if you want (half cup)

(approximately two tablespoons)

Spinach as little as a baby

Oil made from olives

Herb blend from Italy

(half tablespoon)

Ground black pepper and salt are all that is needed to season this dish.

Steps

Toss the sprouts and vegetables together in a large basin.

Then, in a separate bowl, combine the lime juice, salt, italian herb mix, olive oil, and pepper.

When the salad dressing and the vegetables have been combined, you can serve the salad.

10. Chickpea and Kale Mash

Even though it has the appearance of Chinese food, this mash of kale and chickpea is not. It's good for you and has a long list of health advantages.

The recipe comprises

3 cloves of garlic, minced

Shoulder of white onion, or 1 shallot

Kale in a bunch

Cooked chickpeas: 12 cup

Use two tablespoons of coconut oil in this recipe.

a pinch of Celtic sea salt

Steps

After chopping and frying the shallot, you add some minced garlic to the pan.

Add the onion, garlic, and kale after it has been fried till golden brown.

The chickpeas should be cooked for around six minutes.

Toss everything together and enjoy!

Now that you've finished your dish, feel free to dig in.

Warm Oatmeal with a Splash of Vanilla

When it comes to breakfast, there's no better option than cold oatmeal. Make some at home, it's a great way to start the day because it makes you feel and remain cool.

Recipe

Oats, about 12 cup

Skimmed milk in a half-cup measure

The equivalent of half a cup of yoghurt

RECIPES

Cinnamon in a quarter teaspoonful

sliced half a banana

Peanut butter, about a half-worth cup's

Berries: 12 cup of them

Getting Ready

To make it, all you have to do is combine the oats, yoghurt, milk, and salt in a glass jar, and then store it in the refrigerator.

Seal the jar and place it in the refrigerator for the next 24 hours to chill.

In the morning, you can add berries, bananas, and cinnamon.

Chapter Four

My personal recipes

12th Theplas

It is a food that is popular in Gujarat, India, and it is high in fibre. You can substitute it for ordinary oats and it's both nutritious and delicious.

Recipe

fenugreek stems and foliage

A quarter of a cup

One minced clove of garlic

spinach

(equivalent to one-half cup)

The equivalent of 112 mugs

oats with wheat flour

gluten free chickpea starch

The equivalent of 112 mugs

Salt, tumeric, and a dash of pepper.

A little water to help with the dough kneading

Use 2 teaspoons of olive oil in the dough.

It also contains 4 tablespoons of cooking oil

Getting Ready

Fenugreek leaves, salt, turmeric, and water should be added to the flour mixture.

Heat the oil for two minutes in a pan.

Stir in the onions until they begin to acquire a golden brown colour.

Let it cool down before removing it from the heat and adding the spinach.

Knead in the spinach after it has been cooked.

Make little balls out of the dough and place them on a baking sheet. A rolling pin can be used to cut out little circles of the dough.

Thepla should be cooked for two minutes on each side in a hot skillet.

Ten seconds on each side with a teaspoon of oil added.

Serve it while it's still warm!

Porridge made with 13 grammes of maple syrup and millet.

Millet porridge is a great source of protein and amino acids, making it an excellent breakfast option. As far as healthy breakfasts go, these should be on your list of options.

Recipe

2 tablespoons of oats

4 mugs of h2o.

Some salt will go a long way

Cinnamon powder in 1 tbsp

Maple syrup is available in a variety of flavours and strengths.

Getting Ready

To begin, bring a large saucepan of water to a boil. Add salt and millet to the pot while it is still hot. Cook for around 15 minutes with the lid on and the heat lowered. Cook the millets for an additional 20 minutes after adding the cinnamon and almond water. Once you've added the maple syrup, whisk it into the mixture you've already created. Your food is ready when you've done everything you can to get the thickness just right.

Chickpea Frittata is the thirteenth recipe on this list.

The chickpea frittata has the potential to be a fantastic egg frittata replacement for vegans. Both the taste and the nutritional value of this dish are excellent.

The ingredients for this dish are listed below.

Chickpea flour is 1 cup.

1 cup of water

a pound of sliced zucchini

12 cup finely minced onions

12 tsp. ground pepper

A total of 4 tbsp olive oil

Grated garlic from a single clove

Chopped spring onions: 12 cups

Tasty seasoning

Getting Ready

The oven should be preheated at 190 degrees Celsius.

A baking pan or tray should be sprayed with cooking spray or butter.

All save the oil and spring onions should be added to a big bowl before the rest of the ingredients (do not add the oil or spring onions by accident).

Large batch of batter should have 1-2 teaspoons of oil added.

Make sure the pan is well-greased.

Bake for 30 to 45 minutes.

Remove it from the oven and chop it up.

Servants can add spring onions as a garnish.

Recipes for smoothies

In fact, smoothies are calming and can help you maintain muscle mass as you age. Additionally, it can help lower your risk of diabetes while also boosting your immune system. It may also help lower your risk of developing other chronic diseases including heart disease and osteoporosis, as well as cancer.

If you'd like to learn how to "do your own thing" on a diet, you can experiment with different items and determine what works best for you.

The alkaline energy booster smoothie is the first option.

Kale is a key ingredient in this alkaline smoothie, which is quick and easy to prepare and will give you plenty of energy throughout the day. An excellent source of antioxidants, Kale is one of the world's most nutrient dense foods. Heart and cancer-preventive properties are among its many advantages. Strawberries and raspberries have been shown to enhance concentration and short-term memory. I bet you have no idea that berry fruits alter the way neurons communicate. This alteration in the way neurons communicate has a positive effect on brain power.

Requirements

Calf, about 1 cup

The fruit of one banana

Strawberries in half a cup

2 tablespoons of honey

14 cup fresh raspberries

Getting Ready

Fresh or frozen strawberries, bananas, and raspberries can be used. In order to make it more refreshing, the ingredients should be blended in a blender with only a few ice cubes.

Smoothie with alkaline greens

It's awe inspiring! This nutritious and delectable smoothie may be made with only a few simple ingredients. Kale and spinach, when eaten together, can help boost your immune system while also protecting you from cancer. This alkalizing smoothie, made from two powerful superfoods, can help lower your blood pressure and potentially protect you from heart disease. In addition, it's a good source of a variety of essential nutrients.

Requirements

2 cups of spinach

1 bunch of kale

1/3 of a cup of apple cider vinegar

Lemon juice, a single teaspoonful

One-half of a cucumber

Getting Ready

A medium-sized cucumber would be ideal for this recipe. This can be done with either standard or baby spinach. Organic apple juice is recommended for this dish. All of the ingredients must be thoroughly blended.

The berry alkaline smoothie is a very remarkable drink.

This is the ideal smoothie to make when you're short on time but still need to get some nutrition in. Strawberries mixed in a smoothie will keep your mind bright and your body energised. Adding to the benefits, chia seeds are one of the world's healthiest plant foods. They're rich with magnesium, calcium, and manganese, as well as an incredibly low calorie count.

Included in the list of requirements are

Blueberries, around a cup's worth

a single lime

chia seeds, 1 heaping tablespoon

Strawberries in half a cup

Spinach, about a cupful

1 cinnamon stick, ground

One and a half bananas

1/4 of a pint of coconut milk

Getting Ready

Easy to make, despite having more ingredients than the last recipe. Blend the lime juice with the rest of the ingredients in a blender, including the frozen strawberries and the fresh blueberries, if you choose.

Alkaline post-workout shake

Having a post-workout alkaline smoothie provides a wealth of benefits. Mixing almond milk and butter is essential for replenishing energy levels. This macronutrient is critical for muscle recovery and should be consumed as soon as possible following a workout. For a healthier alternative, try avocados, which are rich in healthy fats and can improve the absorption of fat-soluble nutrients.

Requirements

A single avocado

Raw almond butter: 1 tbsp

a litre of almond milk per person

The fruit of one banana

chia seeds in a single tablespoon

Getting Ready

If you want coconut or hemp milk instead of almond, you can do so. The banana should be peeled or frozen, and the rest of the ingredients should be blended until smooth.

Green smoothie with peaches and spinach, high in alkaline

In addition to being one of the most popular summer fruits, peaches are well-known for their sweetness. This fruit has a lot of nutrients in it, therefore it provides a variety of health benefits when consumed. They also have remarkable anti-aging properties due to the zinc they contain. This food contains a lot of vitamin C and other minerals that are good for bones and teeth health. Vitamin C is a powerful immune system booster. In contrast, parsley has been shown to enhance bone health, improve cardiovascular health, and reduce cancer risk.

Requirements

Peaches, 14 cup

a half cup of spinach.

Cucumber, one and a half

Use one fourth-cup-full to garnish

Bananas are available for purchase.

Water in a half cup

a quarter of a lemon

Getting Ready

Squeezing a medium-sized lemon half and pouring the juice into a cup is all you need to do to make this at home. Before putting the peaches in the blender, make sure they are sliced thinly. You need to add a few ice cubes before blending everything together.

Alkaline blueberry smoothie heaven

For all their nutritional value, blueberries are underappreciated because of their relative lack of popularity. Because it contains the antioxidant anthocyanin, it has a wide range of health advantages. Among the many chronic diseases that blueberries help prevent include diabetes, cancer, heart disease, and others due to their high antioxidant content. They will also help you achieve your weight loss objectives since they will make you feel full for a longer period of time, making you less likely to overeat. Because of its high fibre content, this fruit helps you feel fuller for longer.

Requirements

Blueberries, around a cup's worth

Raw almond butter: 1 tbsp

1 spinach leaf

1/4 cup chia seed powder

Ground flax seed: 1 tablespoon

1/4 of a cup of coconut water

a spoonful of organic coconut oil.

The powdered hemp seed is 1 tablespoon.

Getting Ready

The smoothie is ready to be made by simply blending all of the ingredients together. You can simply substitute hemp milk for the coconut milk if you like.

The alkaline smoothie, which has anti-inflammatory properties.

The anti-inflammatory smoothie should be consumed on a regular basis, according to the experts' recommendations.

After five full days, we're done. Omega-3 fatty acids, found in abundance in flax seeds, have been shown to have potent anti-inflammatory effects. Omega-3 fatty acids, such as alpha-linoleic acid, are abundant in flax seeds and have a positive impact on cardiovascular health. Flax seeds are noteworthy for being a very good source of lignin. The substances in these plants are so potent that they may potentially help reduce the risk of cancer.

Requirements

The fruit of one banana

1/4 of a pint of coconut milk

1 tsp. of ground ginger

1 cinnamon stick, ground

Strawberries in half a cup

Calf, about 1 cup

1/2 cup ground flaxseed

Getting Ready

You may make a smoothie by mixing all the ingredients in a blender and blending until smooth. Any other kind of berry can be used in place of the strawberries. Instead of kale, try using a cup of spinach.

Smoothie made with spinach and strawberries

You'll be able to stay energised all day long thanks to this delightful beverage. Spinach's dark, leafy greens (like those in kale) are crucial to bone health, digestive health, and blood pressure reduction as well. Antioxidant-rich strawberries can guard you against a wide range of ailments and diseases.

Requirements

2 mugs of slaw

Strawberries in half a cup

a single lime

The fruit of one banana

1/4 of a pint of coconut milk

Hemp seeds, 1 heaping tablespoon

Getting Ready

It's as simple as that! Make a smooth sauce by combining all of the ingredients in a blender and blending until well combined. The banana can either be fresh or frozen, but you must squeeze the lime juice out of it before putting it in the blender. Even if the smoothie is already sweet, you can sweeten it further using stevia.

Smoothie with Kiwi and Cucumber

You can't help but fall in love with kiwi because of its flavour. In addition to its exquisite flavour, kiwi is an extremely nutritious fruit. Oxidative damage to your cell DNA can be prevented by eating this fruit. Additionally, the immune system can be bolstered and your blood pressure can be regulated as a result of this fruit. Hydration, weight loss, and cardiovascular health are all supported by cucumber. When these two come together, you have a strong team.

Requirements

A single kiwi fruit

A quarter of a cucumber

One and a half bananas

1 spinach leaf

Three to four almonds

A quarter cup of coconut milk

Getting Ready

A blender is all you need to make this, and you can even add a few ice cubes to the blender to make it more refreshing.

Breakfast smoothie with alkaline minerals

In addition to being one of the greatest weight loss smoothies, this one is delicious and refreshing. Grapefruits, which are abundant in antioxidants like beta-carotene, vitamin C, and lycopene, and are known to promote satiety, may help you cut calories. Collard greens, on the other hand, may assist in the process of detoxification while also improving the appearance of your skin. They also have the ability to reduce cholesterol levels. In order to really lower your cholesterol levels, you need eat some of these.

Requirements

Two grapes

3-foot-long collard greens

A little over one cup of pomegranate arils

1/4 of a pint of coconut milk

Getting Ready

The grapefruits must first be peeled, and the seeds must be removed. Collard leaves' stems must also be cut off. It's time to combine the components, so do that now. To make it sweeter, you may add a little stevia.

Recipes for a Light Lunch

Trying to figure out what to eat for lunch may be a difficult task, and eating the same thing over and over again is a bad idea. If you're following an alkaline diet, it can be difficult to know what to eat for lunch after you've had your morning meal.

While it's tempting to just eat what you had for breakfast and call it a day, this isn't the healthiest option as we need to eat three meals a day nevertheless. They each play a specific job in ensuring that the body functions optimally.

Here are some lunchtime recipes that are quick to make and may be kept on hand at all times.

Sushi made with zucchini

This is one of the best lunches you can make, yet it doesn't involve a lot of time or work. The zucchini sushi

Included among the ingredients are

2 medium-sized courgettes

4 ounces of softened cream cheese

Sriracha hot sauce, 1 tsp.

a tablespoon of lime juice.

1 oz. of lump crab.

a quarter of a carrot, thinly sliced

12 an avocado, sliced finely

A matchstick-thin half of a cucumber.

Sesame seeds, heated till fragrant, 1 teaspoon

Getting Ready

Slice the zucchini into thin, flat strips and set aside on a platter lined with paper towels while the rest of the ingredients are made.

In a medium bowl, combine the cream cheeses, sriracha, and lime juice.

A horizontal arrangement of two zucchini slices is depicted (make the long side to face you). To begin, a layer of cream cheese should be put on top, followed by a layer of crab, avocado, and cucumber on the left side.

The zucchini should be folded up starting from the left side. Using the remaining zucchini slices and filling, repeat this process. Before serving, top with a few sesame seeds. That is all there is to it!

The Citrus Vinaigrette Salad:

Among them are the following: (Salad)

1-inch-long julienned zucchini, one and a half cups

Julienned squash, equal to the amount listed in the previous step.

maize kernels, 1 cup (must be fresh, about 2 ears)

12 cups julienned red peppers (1 inch long)

Red onions, coarsely chopped, 3 teaspoons

finely chopped 2 tblsp. flat leaf parsley

1 tablespoon of freshly chopped fresh basil

What's in it? (vinaigrette)

The juice of three oranges is enough for this recipe.

a half-cup of freshly squeezed lime juice

Olive oil, extra virgin, 3 tbsp

Honey in the amount of 2-3 tablespoons

1 tsp. of vinegar made from red wine

The equivalent of a quarter teaspoon of sea salt

The equivalent of 1/8th of a black peppercorn

Getting Ready (salad)

Combine the zucchini and all other ingredients in a big bowl to make the salad.

Preparation is key (vinaigrette)

All you have to do is combine everything and give it a good swirl. Toss the salad with the vinaigrette, then cover and refrigerate.

So there you have it, a fantastic lunch!

Chickpeas with honey sesame flavour

These are some of the most mouth-watering foods on the face of the planet. Alkaline diet foods have all the nutrients necessary for a healthy diet, and more. They keep the body well-nourished and hydrated.

Included among the ingredients are

Finely sliced onion, about 1 small cup

The minced garlic of two cloves

Honey in half a cup.

a tbsp. of oyster sauce

Toasted sesame oil in 2 tablespoons.

Vinegar made with rice wine

The oil is 2 tablespoons

water, 14 cup

4 milligrammes of ground cayenne pepper

1 tsp. fresh ginger root grated

Chickpeas

Cooked dry chickpeas, drained and rinsed, one and a half cups

Rice that has been cooked and is ready to be served.

Getting Ready

In a medium saucepan, combine the finely chopped onion, minced garlic, sesame oil, vinegar, vegetable oil, honey soy sauce, red pepper flakes, and ginger. The sauce should be brought to a boil, then simmered for 5 to 10 minutes, or until it is slightly thickened (about 14 cup thick).

Once the chickpeas have been added, the mixture should be brought back to a rolling boil. Simmer for another 10 minutes until the chickpeas are coated and the sauce thickens, then remove from the heat.

Serve the honey sesame chickpeas over hot cooked rice, and do it as soon as possible after preparing them.

The same sesame seeds and cut scallions should be used for the garnish (this one is optional).

4. The sauce of red cabbage, beetroot, and apple.

The ingredients include

Finely shaved slices of three apples

650 grammes of finely cut red cabbage

Peeled and grated beetroot (250 grammes)

2-teaspoon vinegar, or apple cider

12 a cup of lemon juice

An extra virgin olive oil of 5 tbsp

Seeds from 50 pomegranates

Chopped parsley in a small container

Getting Ready

Mix the vinegar, lemon juice, oil, and seasoning together and pour it over the cabbage mixture before placing it in a big bowl. Before serving, it should be thoroughly combined with the pomegranate and parsley.

Chocolate-coconut-chia bars with toasty coconut flavour

The ingredients include

1 cup of coconut flakes, shredded, unsweetened

3 Medrol dates that have been pitted

Brown rice syrup: 2 teaspoons

Almond butter, two tablespoons

1 tbsp. chocolate chips, miniature

Water, one-and-a-half tablespoons (if there is any need)

Getting Ready

Toasting shredded coconut in a pan over medium heat is the best way to do it. Until the coconut flakes get golden, keep tossing them. It should just take a few minutes to complete this. Just keep an eye on it, since you don't want to burn the coconut. Allow the coconut to cool for about ten minutes after it has been removed from the fire.

In a food processor, combine the toasted coconut that has been allowed to cool, along with dates, brown rice syrup, chia seeds, almond butter, and chocolate chips. Process until a dough-like consistency begins to form. If the mixture is too dry and doesn't form a ball, a small amount of water (approximately one and a half tablespoons) can be added.

Remove the dough from the processor and push it onto a parchment-lined 8-inch loaf pan. To help the bars harden, the loaf pan should be placed in the refrigerator for 30 to 60 minutes. Cut it into six bars and keep it in the refrigerator until you're hungry.

6. Butternut squash soup with a creamy sauce.

The ingredients include

14 cup finely diced onions

This recipe calls for a teaspoonful of butter.

3 cups of diced butternut squash, cleaned and drained

Chopped up a medium-sized potato

a cup to a cup and a half

1-2 tablespoons of chicken bouillon granules per quart of water

14 tsp. of sea salt

Add a pinch of cayenne pepper

One-fourth cup of evaporation milk

Getting Ready

In a small saucepan, cook the onion until softened with the butter. Cook and toss the squash and potato for about 2 minutes. Bring to a boil the water, bouillon, salt, and pepper. Cover and boil the vegetables for about 15 to 20 minutes, or until they're fork-tender.

Allow it to cool a bit. Blend the soup in a blender until it is completely smooth. Pour the mixture back into the pan, add the milk, and bring it to a boil.

Vegetable soup with a rich broth

The ingredients include

Carrots chopped into eight medium-size pieces.

2 big onions finely sliced

Celery ribs that have been finely sliced

Seeded and diced up one large green pepper

a teaspoon of olive oil

1 minced clove of garlic

4 mugs of h2o.

2 cups chopped tomatoes, undrained

Juice from two cans of V8

Chopped cabbage: 2 cups.

Cut green beans, 2 cups, from the frozen section

Frozen peas in 2 quarts

1 cup of corn, defrosted

Rinse and drain a can of garbanzo beans or chickpeas before using.

2 teaspoons of granulated chicken bouillon

Dried parsley flakes can be used in place of fresh parsley.

a sprinkling of salt

Dried marjoram is one teaspoon.

Dried thyme, one teaspoon.

one bay leaf

Dry basil, one-half teaspoon

14 tsp. ground pepper

Getting Ready

Using medium heat, sauté carrots and celery, onions and green pepper in a stockpot with the oil until they are soft and translucent. Then, add the garlic and heat and stir for a further one minute. As you bring the rest of the ingredients to a boil, stir them in.

The temperature should be lowered, then simmered and covered until the vegetables are soft. An hour and a half would be ideal for this task. After that, remove the bay leaf from the bowl.

Lemon vinaigrette-smothered Kale and Quinoa Salad

The ingredients include (kale and quinoa salad)

1 cup of quinoa that has been well washed

2 quarts of fluid

2 cups of loosely packed, finely chopped kale

Dried cranberries or raisins, half a cup

walnuts, diced, half a cup

The ingredients include (Lemon vinaigrette)

Olive oil, unrefined and undiluted, 1/4 cup

Freshly squeezed lemon juice in equal parts

Salt from the ocean, 1/8 tsp.

a teaspoon of mustard seed

Dried oregano in a quarter teaspoon

The equivalent of 1/8th of a black peppercorn

Getting Ready

Toss the walnuts with the quinoa after it has been cooked for 10 minutes on a baking pan and roast for another 10 minutes at 325 degrees. Allow it to cool and then put it aside.

To prepare the salad, place the quinoa in a medium saucepan and bring to a boil over medium-high heat, stirring occasionally. When the quinoa has absorbed most of the liquid, decrease the heat to a medium-simmer, cover, and cook for about 15 minutes. After the heat has been turned off, add the kale and cranberries to the pot. When the kale has wilted, the covered pot should be left on the burner for roughly 7 minutes.

All components for the lemon vinaigrette should be put in a glass container and whisked until smooth. Before serving, let it sit in the refrigerator for at least an hour or two.

Cooking Ideas for Dinner

Nowadays, eating healthfully is more than just a fad. Health experts from across the world are hard at work conducting studies to determine the best ways to live a healthy lifestyle. The opposite is also true: they're finding better ways to stay healthy, lose weight, and maintain a healthy level of acidity in the body. Eating healthily is a simple matter of knowing what to cook and what to consume. For a healthy lifestyle, the alkaline diet offers a wide variety of dietary options.

Here are some alkaline diet dinner recipes that are both nutritious and easy to prepare in less than five minutes. If you're on the run and don't have much time to make a healthy alkaline food, this is a godsend for you.

Spread made with avocado and green peas:

Intensely flavorful green pea and avocado toasts. It has a pleasant and refreshing flavour, with a hint of green peas and avocado mixed in. This can serve as a dip for your best vegetables, it can function as a salad scoop and you can add it to a wrapper. In addition to being a healthful recipe, this one is extremely versatile. To make the green pea and avocado spread, gather the following ingredients:

two servings of green peas, either fresh or frozen

1 pitted and roughly cut mini avocado

3 tablespoons of finely chopped green onion or chives

Two-and-a-half tablespoons

1,4,and1,8

Eat a lot of raw and leafy greens

The most crucial aspect of this is that almost all leafy green vegetables may be eaten raw. If that's not your cup of tea, you can always prepare a salad by blending together a variety of leafy greens and calling it a day. Now you've got a quick, healthy, and delicious alkaline dish that just takes five minutes to prepare.

There is nothing else that is as simple and quick to put together as a meal. Kale, spinach, romaine, cabbage, mustard greens, broccoli, avocado, and celery are just a few of the vegetables you can use in this recipe. There are no restrictions on the kind of leafy greens you can eat.

Your salad might be more appealing and pleasant for you by adding a little bit of spice. When food isn't well-dressed or designed, many people find it tedious. Add some fresh garlic, tomatoes, radishes, fresh thyme, basil, and mint to your veggie salad to make it more visually appealing. Perhaps some peppers would be a good addition if they aren't enough for you. Any colour peppers can be used, including green, yellow, and red peppers.

Adding a squeeze of lime or lemon, or substituting apple cider vinegar for some other acidic dressings, is another option.

However, there are many more veggies that can be considered, and they all have some alkalinity in them. When it comes to combining these fruits and vegetables to create a healthy alkaline diet, your lack of imagination is largely to blame for this problem. In fact, most of them are extremely alkaline in nature.

Vegetables that have been boiled:

It's only natural that some people prefer their vegetables to be softer to eat, in the same way that salad dressing and vegetables go together. You don't have to rely just on salads when it comes to preparing your leafy greens for an alkaline meal.

Try steaming your vegetables if raw vegetables or salads don't work for you. In certain cases, like broccoli and cauliflower, consumers prefer them softer, so they can quickly steam them to their preferred texture before eating.

Asparagus, green beans, and Brussels sprouts are some examples of vegetables that can be steamed or roasted before being eaten.

It's hard to forget about tuber foods such as new potatoes, which are one of the most alkaline-friendly tubers. Carrots, sweet potatoes, peas, and squash are just a few of the numerous tuber vegetables you can and should eat in your alkaline diet plan.

These tuber veggies are incredibly filling thanks to their solid texture. For a long period, they can keep you from needing to eat any additional food. Consider adding leeks, eggplants, beets, and zucchini to the mix. This is an excellent alkaline diet recipe because it's simple and fast to make.

Smoothie with blackberries:

A blender makes it a lot simpler to make smoothies. Yes, you can make smoothies with a blender. If you have a blender, you can make and have that smoothie whenever you want. If you don't already have a blender in your kitchen, you might want to acquire one now. Having a decent blender is essential. Without the blender, there will be no smoothie.

For an alkaline diet meal, blackberry smoothies are a great choice. To prepare a blackberry smoothie, combine 1 12 cups of coconut milk with a bunch of dark leafy greens in a blender. The blender will then be filled with the following ingredients:

- 1 cup of blackberries, thawed

frozen strawberries, about 12 oz.

- 1 lime that has been squeezed to its full potential

Two teaspoons of coconut oil is all you need.

- 2 drops of Medicine Flower Vanilla, or a half-teaspoon

Additionally, you can add a spoonful of raw almond butter to your smoothie.

Blackberries are a great source of calcium for the body, which is why they're so popular. This combination will help your bones stay strong, battle acidity in the body, and nourish your entire body at the same time. This recipe is extremely potent because of this. In addition to this, blackberry smoothies contain a wide range of flavours, making them a great alkaline combo.

Coconut milk that does not include preservatives or additives is a good choice for an alkaline diet, according to this tiny hint. Having merely coconut and water in a coconut milk is a real treat.

Millet:

The great alkaline components of millet make it an excellent addition to an alkaline diet.

Below, we've included some of millet's incredible advantages and some things you should know about millet:

There are several varieties of millet, a type of small seeded grasses that are farmed all over the world for human use. Pennisetum glaucum, often known as pearl millet, is the most prevalent type of millet in the world.

Millets can be used as local cereals, but they can also be used to make porridge, bread, and snacks.

Foods rich in carbohydrates as well as fibre, such as millets, can be found here. Millet is also a good source of vitamins and nutrients as well as minerals and other organic substances, all of which have a positive impact on human health.

Grain products free of gluten should include millets. It's for the benefit of those who experience responses to certain gluten-containing celiac meals. As a result, millet consumption serves as a substitute for celiac diets while avoiding celiac illness. Millets are a good source of energy, lipids, and vitamin B; they're also a good source of fibre.

Vitamin B, iron, potassium, calcium, magnesium and zinc are all found in significant concentrations in millets. They also have a high degree of dietary fibre. Millet's nutritional value is enhanced by a wide range of factors, including these.

Millets have also been shown to reduce the risk of heart disease over time. Millets, on the other hand, may be a good option if you wish to protect your heart. Magnesium is abundant in millets. For the decrease of blood pressure, the risk of heart disease and stroke, particularly in the context of atherosclerosis, magnesium is essential.

Millets are also abundant in potassium, which serves as a vasodilator and lowers blood pressure. You can avoid heart disease if you keep your cholesterol levels in check. Because high cholesterol is often a contributing factor to heart disease.

Millet is a good source of dietary fibre, and this is one of its benefits.

Because they don't contain gluten, millets are an uncommon grain. It is high in fibre and low in glycemic index, making it a good source of both. This has a favourable effect on diabetes, in particular. Millets are also helpful in preventing and slowing the spread of diabetes over the globe.

Digestion, elimination of constipation, bloating and other gas and bloating issues, detoxification, the prevention of asthma and cramps are all benefits of eating millets. In addition to these benefits, millet is a suitable choice for alkaline diets because of its high fibre content. Millet is in the grain family, and some grain items aren't great for everyone. If you've never tried millet, this might be a good time.

Millet is a tasty treat if you enjoy sweets. Millets have a flavour that is a cross between sweet and nutty. Other beneficial chemical compounds and vitamins abound in this superfood. In addition, it provides the body with protein.

Millets can be used to produce porridge, snack bread, and sweet bread. Millet, on the other hand, may be used in a variety of ways and has a high value. Due of its many established uses, including in almost any type of dish that employs rice or quinoa, this is why. For soups and stews, it can also be used as stuffing or as a casserole. In order to improve the taste, because it may be pretty bland, you may need some really good spices and herbs to make it taste the way you want. While serving, cinnamon and diced fruits can be added.

Millet is a simple and straightforward dish to prepare. All you need to get started is a cup of millet, 2 and 12 glasses of water, and approximately a half a teaspoon of sea salt. To avoid overcooking or undercooking, cook it over a medium heat until it reaches a golden brown colour, then mix it regularly to achieve the appropriate texture.

Wraps made from vegetables:

Alkaline diet dishes can not get much easier than this one. All you need for a vegetable wrap is some chopped vegetables and a large amount of leafy greens to wrap them in. Preservative and less time-consuming, a vegetable wrap is a great option. As a result, you're free to reuse and recycle any leftovers. You can build a veggie wrap with your leftovers and some other ingredients to give it a more fresh and colourful appearance; hummus is an option to explore. Making a large number of veggie wraps only takes a few minutes, maybe even five.

Beans and zucchini: Any form of cooked bean goes well with any type of zucchini. Isn't that incredible? Zucchini, whether conventional or spiralized, can be served with a variety of prepared beans. There is nothing complicated about them; all you have to do is cook them in grass-fed or coconut or ghee butter. Zucchinis can be prepared in a variety of ways.

Zucchini can be prepared in a variety of ways to achieve the flavour you like. Zucchini can be spiced up with the addition of herbs like basil or thyme, as well as garlic or cumin. Zucchini is a versatile vegetable that can be flavoured and tasted according to individual preferences. You have complete control over the flavourings that go into your food preparation. In addition to that, don't forget to stir-fry. To speed up the process of cooking your beans, you should stir-fry them together with any additional ingredients you think may help. It's easy to make a variety of zucchini and bean dishes, and the results are both delicious and nutritious.

Zucchinis are quick and simple to prepare, taking no more than a few minutes from start to finish.

With Brussels sprouts, lemon, and pistachios, this dish comes together quickly and easily.

Adding pistachios, lemon, and Brussels sprouts to your diet will make you feel full and satisfied for hours. Brussels sprouts can also be prepared in a short amount of time. Below you'll find the ingredients and directions for creating it yourself.

In a skillet or wok, melt 2 tablespoons of grass-fed butter.

Pistachios, lemon zest, and at least a minute of cooking are all that's needed after that.

Add 16 Brussels sprout leaves to the sauté and continue tossing until the Brussels sprout gets a vibrant green hue. This should take you around five minutes to complete.

With the lemon still in your hand, squeeze its juice over the Brussels sprouts and pistachios. Season with salt and pepper if needed. If you choose, you can also add some herbs to it.

As a reminder, this quick and easy meal is packed with nutrients such as vitamin C, minerals and alkalinity.

a salad of avocadoes with red onion and tomatoes:

Looking at the combo, you can see right away that it's packed with nutrition. That's a potent mix, isn't it? Without a doubt, the nutrients in this dish will satisfy your hunger. When it comes to making an Avocado tomato and red onion salad, how do you go about it? Ahead of us:

Get a couple of avocados and cut them into cubes.

Season it with a dash of salt and pepper, if desired.

Add half an onion and a chopped tomato to a different bowl. You can also add the other half of a jalapeño pepper and stir it all together before serving.

Add a quarter cup of finely chopped cilantro or parsley to this mixture.

Lemon juice and extra virgin olive oil should be added to the mixture.

Lastly, add one tea spoon of cumin.

Now combine them with the avocados.

Oleic acid, which is naturally present in avocadoes, makes you feel full and fulfilled, making them an excellent source of vitamins and minerals. Avocados also include cilantro, a heavy metal purgative herb that aids the body in combating and eliminating pollutants.

Due to the quercitin found in both yellow and red pepper, it is beneficial for decreasing cholesterol levels, thinning the blood, and combating both infections and atherosclerosis. You can see that this is a great alkaline diet meal to have on hand at any time. If you eat this late at night, you can go to sleep knowing you've had one of the healthiest meals you've ever had. You will undoubtedly awaken with a positive outlook on your physical appearance and self-esteem.

a glass of water flavoured with fresh lemon juice:

Lemon water, that's right. Lemon should be your go-to thirst-quencher instead of sodas and pop. In terms of health benefits, it is far superior to sugar-sweetened beverages like sodas and pop. To make lemonade, all you have to do is like lemonade because everyone likes lemonade! Sugar is the only thing missing from this recipe. This recipe does not include any sugar and never will.

In two to four glasses of water, add the squeezed juice of a cut lemon. The taste of stevia can be substituted for sugar. Stevia is a wonderful sugar replacement. There will be no sweeteners in this recipe. Processed sugar is often discouraged by nutritionists. So, don't try to get away with adding some fake sugar to get a better deal.

If you're curious about whether lemons have an acidic flavour, the answer is yes, as they do. However, despite their acidic flavour, they are digested and broken down as alkaline in the body. Lemons are safe to eat, as long as you don't eat too many. Taking a glass of lemon water is also a wonderful idea. Vitamin C and B6 are found in high concentrations in lemons. All of these nutrients may be found in lemons as well, as well as potassium. That already has the potential to sound fantastic!

The best part about making alkaline cuisine is that it doesn't need a lot of time or effort. It's neither long-lasting nor difficult to perform. The alkaline food plan is just as adaptable as other acidic meal plans. There are countless alkaline dishes that are beneficial to your health and nutrition. The minerals, vitamins, and other nutrients that they provide can help your body battle pollutants and detoxify at the same time.

Another alkaline diet meal for a good dinner is spelt porridge. The steps and ingredients needed to create spelt porridge that will serve at least two people are listed below.

Ingredients:

- Filtered water (two cups)

- 2/3 cup spelt flaked thin

- Cinnamon powder (this is for taste)

- Agave syrup (for taste); powdered stevia can be substituted for agave syrup.

- 12 tea spoon vanilla extract (use alcohol-free vanilla extract)

- 4–6 teaspoons dried cherries or cranberries

Some people like to customise their own pizza, which is quite OK. You can use any of the following toppings as a garnish:

- Strawberries, blackberries, blueberries, seeds, hemp nuts, raw nuts, or fresh raspberries are all good options.

- 1 cup hemp, 1 cup rice milk, 1 cup unsweetened almond or hazel nut

Prepare it as follows:

- Return to the original list and combine the first six components.

- Set the heat to medium and cook the mixture for at least three to four minutes.

- Pour it into a large mixing bowl.

- If you have any advantages, scatter them around the top of the mixture.

- Pour some non-dairy milk over it.

- You can eat your spelt porridge now.

Smoothies with coconut water, blueberries, and almond milk:

Coconut water is typically healthy and can be used to create delicious alkaline diet recipes. Here's how to prepare a smoothie using coconut water, almond milk, and blueberries.

Ingredients:

- 1 cup almond milk (unsweetened)

- Blueberries (two cups) (best to use frozen one)

- 2 1/2 cups coconut water

- One and a third cup raspberries (best to use frozen own)

- Avocados (two)

- 4 teaspoons agave syrup or 4 teaspoons xylitol

- 6 table spoons coconut flesh
- 2 tea spoons pure vanilla powder (or alcohol-free vanilla liquid)
- Super greens powder (one to two tea spoons)
- 4 teaspoons omega-3 oil
- Raw hemp nuts (six to eight table spoons)

How to Get Ready:

- Combine all ingredients in a blender.
- Blend thoroughly to finely mince the raspberry seeds.
- If extra coconut water is required for consistency, do so.

Spread with cannellini beans and artichokes:

Another amazing alkaline supper meal. Here are the ingredients and techniques for preparing a cannellini bean and artichoke spread.

Ingredients:

- 2 garlic cloves, roughly chopped
- 2 shallots, roughly chopped
- 4 teaspoons lemon juice
- Lemon zest (two tea spoons)
- 2/3 cup extra virgin olive oil

- Two cannellini beans, rinsed and drained (preferable to use organic)
- 2 tins artichoke hearts, bottoms, and drained organic artichoke
- 12 tea spoons of salt
- 12 tea spoon pepper, freshly ground
- Tarragon leaves, approximately 24

How to Get Ready:

- In a food processor, combine the ingredients.
- Make certain you combine them.
- Turn the processor off and pickle the insides of a bowl.
- Re-blend the mixture until it is completely mixed.
- Add extra oil if necessary to get a spreadable consistency.
- Season with salt to enhance flavour.

Soup with vegetables:

A good alkaline diet recipe is an organic soup. What could be better than a steaming bowl of organic soup? Alkaline diets contain the proper recipes for you, whatever you want.

Here's everything you'll need to prepare a hearty vegetable soup:

- 12 onion bulb, diced
- 1 garlic clove, crumpled or minced
- One and a half big carrots, chopped
- 1 1/2 pound chopped potatoes

Rice balls and spinach with a high protein content:

Making these is both enjoyable and simple. Forget about the green; youngsters will like it as well. These also freeze nicely, allowing them to be prepared ahead of time and kept for later consumption. You can simply take them out whenever you want and reheat them in the oven before serving. The centre of the rice balls and the outside of the protein spinach are soft and crispy. They're also high in protein and help with iron absorption.

Below is a recipe for rice balls with protein spinach:

Ingredients:

- 4 & 1/2 cup spinach leaves
- a third of a cup of pitted Greek olives
- 1 teaspoon of nutritional yeast
- 1 teaspoon lemon juice
- 1 tablespoon garlic powder
- 34 teaspoon salt

- 1 quart boiled rice

- 12 cup almond powder

- 1 12 cup chickpea flour

You can serve this with coconut yoghurt or cashew sour cream on top.

How to Get Ready:

- Preheat the oven to approximately 360 degrees Fahrenheit.

- In a food processor, combine the first six ingredients and process until smooth.

- Pour the mixture into a large mixing basin and stir in the remaining three ingredients. Turn them well until a beautiful dough-like texture emerges. If it turns out to be too wet, add a little more chickpea flour to hold the dough together.

- Season with pepper if desired, but avoid tasting it because uncooked chickpeas are bitter.

- Roll it into 12 balls with your hands and place them on a baking sheet. It's usually a jumble, but that's part of the pleasure. Always remember to use baking paper to line your baking tray.

- Place it in the preheated oven and bake it. Do this for approximately 20 to 25 minutes.

- Know when you're ready to go when the bitter taste has faded. You can find out by examining or tasting one of the balls.

Greek Spinach Pie (Spanakopita)

For health reasons, some of the classic dish's ingredients have been substituted in this recipe. The spanakopita is a traditional Greek dish, however this recipe is suitable for an alkaline diet.

Ingredients:

- 12 phyllo dough sheets
- 1 cup finely chopped onion
- 1 cup green onion, chopped
- 4 garlic cloves, minced
- 1 (15) can oz. garbanzo beans, mashed after draining, preferably with little or no sodium
- 2 (10) oz. thawed packaged frozen and sliced spinach
- 2 tbsp nutritional yeast
- 1/3 cup kalamata olives, chopped
- a third cup of tahini
- a quarter cup of lemon juice
- 2 table spoons oregano, freshly crushed

- 2 table spoons crushed fresh parsley
- Season with black pepper to taste.
- 4 tblsp. lemon juice (flaxseed mixture)
- 2 tblsp pure maple syrup
- 2 tblsp flax seed meal

How to Get Ready:

- Preheat the oven to 350 degrees Fahrenheit (175 degrees Celsius).

- Spray a baking pan with cooking powder and set it aside.

- In a nonstick skillet, saute the onion, green onion, two table spoons of water, and garlic over medium heat.

- Cook water on medium heat for about 5 minutes, looking periodically to see whether a table spoon of water or so is required to prevent possible stickiness. This should be done until the onions are transparent.

- Add the spinach and cook for another five minutes, or until the extra liquid has evaporated. While the spinach is cooking, combine the remaining lemon juice, maple syrup, and flaxseed meal in a small bowl.

- Stir until thoroughly combined, then set aside to thicken.

- Set aside the phyllo dough and continue to sauté the remaining ingredients for another five minutes before placing aside to cool.

- Using a small pastry brush, apply the flaxseed mixture to a sheet of phyllo dough in a baking dish. Repeat with the remaining phyllo sheets, then pour the mixture into the pan.

- Bake for 30 to 40 minutes in a preheated oven, until golden brown, then remove from oven and cut into squares.

Recipes for Dessert

Alkaline-based meals are endless, which means there are a million and one recipes and preparation methods. Alkaline diet recipes span a wide spectrum, whether you're seeking for a very filling meal or something to stimulate your appetite.

Chia pudding with vanilla and coconut:

This takes around ten minutes to prepare and should be made the night before to keep in the fridge until the next day. Chia was employed for vitality and strength in Mayan and Aztec cultures due to its 50 percent omega 3 concentration. This is one of the most abundant sources of fatty acids and protein, as well as fibre. All of these properties of Chia make it ideal for healthy cooking. Chia's high fibre content makes it an agent that fights or, more accurately, aids in the reduction of gastrointestinal inflammation. It also helps to decrease cholesterol levels. Chia is high in health-promoting elements, as evidenced by its potential to aid patients suffering from constipation.

Chia contains roughly 18% of your daily calcium, 35% phosphorus, 24% magnesium, and 50% manganese. This is why it is regarded as one of the most effective acid level managers and pH balancers.

To make vanilla coconut chia pudding, follow these steps:

Ingredients:

- 2 cups coconut water (or filtered water if you prefer) Coconut water, however, is sweeter.

- 12 oz. cashews

- 2 tblsp. coconut oil

- 3 dates pitted

- a quarter teaspoon of salt (consider Redmond Real Salt, Celtic Grey, or Himalayan)

- 1 table spoon coconut flakes (unsweetened)

- 2 vanilla tea spoons

- 1 cinnamon tea spoon

- Chia seeds, 6 table spoons

- Consider incorporating cinnamon or pomegranate seeds as a garnish.

How to Get Ready:

- In a blender, combine all ingredients except the Chia seeds and Pomegranate seeds. Blend until everything is thoroughly combined and incorporated.

- After that, add the Chia, but at the slowest speed possible. After mixing for at least one minute, transfer to an airtight container and chill for at least five hours before serving.

- If you want, you can top it with pomegranate seeds or cinnamon. This is also a choice. Other flavours, such as chocolate toppings, can be added before the initial mixture: 14 cup raw cacao. Four to five droplets of nimble chocolate oil taste are also recommended.

- And that's it; dessert is now ready to be served.

Tropical chocolate monkey, frozen:

Ice cream is probably the only, or at least the first, item that comes to mind when you hear the word frozen. But, hey, frozen dessert is so much more than that. You now know that there are numerous frozen delicacies available on a hot day. Frozen chocolate tropical monkey, repeat the name. That's correct, it's frozen, delicious but not too sweet, tropical, and chocolate. Everything you didn't realise you were capable of.

This is fantastic for keeping track of your acidity levels. Despite the lower sugar content, it has a good amount of vitamins and minerals. The banana provides the majority of the sugar. So, instead of using regular sugar, you use sweet organic nutrients like Chia seeds and coconut milk. So there's a sweetness to it, but no acidity.

This is also available to children. How to make chocolate monkeys is as follows:

Ingredients:

- 2 bananas, frozen
- 2 tblsp. coconut oil
- 2 tblsp. cacao powder
- 1 tblsp. cacao nibs
- 2 teaspoons chia seeds

2 quarts coconut milk

How to Get Ready:

- Remove the Chia seeds, pour the remaining ingredients into a blender, and blend until smooth.
- Beat in the Chia seeds one or two times.
- And there you have it: monkey chocolate!

Non-Dairy Berry Parfait

For a healthy diet, try this berry parfait. An iced dish prepared of egg yolks, sugar, cream, and primarily fruit flavouring is known as a parfait. It's a dish that originated in France. The American version is a tiered dessert with fruits, ice cream, pastries, whipped topping, and other ingredients. A parfait is a pate made from liver and flavoured liqueurs in the United Kingdom.

This one is different because it is based on an alkaline eating plan. It's a berry parfait with less dairy items and lower acidity. It has a lot of alkaline elements that balance out the berry's moderate acidity. Combining naturally higher sugar fruits with healthy fats and plant-based proteins is the greatest way to enjoy them. Coconut milk, hemp seed, raw almonds, and cashews come to mind. The beauty of this recipe is that it works well not only as a dessert but also as a breakfast or supper dish, so have fun creating and enjoying it. The supplies and instructions for preparing berry parfaits are as follows:

Ingredients:

- 12 cup cashews, soaking (soak between 20 to 60 minutes.)
- 12 cup almond or coconut milk, unsweetened
- 12 tea spoon vanilla extract (alcohol-free)
- 1 cup berries, frozen
- 1/3 cup gluten-free rolled oats (cooking not required)

1 teaspoon hemp seeds

How to Get Ready:

• To prepare cashew cream, combine cashews, coconut milk, and vanilla in a blender and puree until smooth.

• In a tiny cup, combine your ingredients: a dab of cashew cream, a tablespoon of berries, oats, and hemp seeds, and enjoy.

• And that's it, or as they say, voila! It's time for dessert.

Frozen banana chocolate

This is suitable for both adults and children.

Ingredients:

• 2 bananas, frozen

• 3 table spoons cacao powder (raw)

• 1 table spoon almond butter (raw)

• 14 cup almond milk (unsweetened)

1 teaspoon hemp seeds This is an optional topping.

• 1 table spoon chia seeds (optional and used as a topping)

How to Get Ready:

• Blend the bananas and cacao together in a blender.

- Blend in the almond milk until it reaches the consistency of frozen yoghurt.

- Garnish with chosen seeds and enjoy your chocolate banana fro-yo.

Cookies with organic chocolate chips

This has a very low gluten content, and you may make it with sprouted whole wheat flour. If you don't think you can afford to start sprouting wheat berries or grinding and dehydrating them, that is.

Ingredients:

- spelt flour (14 cup)

- 1 cup whole wheat sprouted floor

- 1 tblsp. baking soda

- 12 tea spoon Himalayan or Celtic sea salt

- 1 cup butter from grass-fed cows

- 1 cup sugar made from coconut palms

- 2 vanilla tea spoons

- 2 eggs

- 34 cup raisins (organic)

- 34 cup coconut flakes or chips

- Chocolate chips that are organic
- 12 cup pecans (this is optional)

How to Get Ready:

- Preheat the oven to 357 degrees Fahrenheit.
- Sift your flour and set it aside with the baking soda and salt.
- In a mixing dish, soften your butter.
- Beat in the coconut palm sugar until it is creamy.
- While mixing, add the eggs and vanilla extract.
- Mix your dry ingredients into a batter until it forms a dough.
- Toss in the coconut chips, chocolate chips, raisins, and nuts, if using. The nuts are not required.
- On a baking sheet, place roughly one or two table spoons of servings.
- Bake for 9 to 12 minutes at 350°F. Allow it to bake until golden brown.

Almond pulp with green apple raw cookies

With this recipe, you can produce a healthy pulp and organic based cookie out of green apples and almonds. The ingredients needed to create one dish are shown below; you can double the recipe to make extra servings.

Ingredients:

- 2 12 to 3 cup almond pulp
- At least seven dates—nine is optional
- 1 apple, granny smith
- 1–12 teaspoons blackstrap molasses
- 1 to 2 cinnamon tea spoons
- 2–3 teaspoons raw honey
- 14 cup coconut flakes, which is optional but takes longer to dehydrate.

How to Get Ready:

- To make a dough, combine all of the ingredients in a food processor and process until a gritty mixture forms that can be cracked into bars or cookies.
- Place the cookies and bars on a baking sheet in a food dehydrator.
- Dehydrate it at 105 to 115 degrees Fahrenheit for 6 to 10 hours, depending on how thick they are.
- Refrigerate for up to 10 days, then enjoy your cookies and pulp.

There are a few more optional ingredients to think about. Ground cloves, cocoa nibs, cocoa powder, almonds, coconut palm sugar, chocolate chips, seeds such as Chia or hemp seeds, and many others are among them.

CPSIA information can be obtained
at www.ICGtesting.com
Printed in the USA
LVHW061207190722
723853LV00014B/549